The Remedy for breast cancer

Step by step measures to conquering breast cancer

By

Linda A. Ivey

Table of content

Introduction

When a malignant (cancerous) tumor develops in the breast, breast cancer results, breast cancer tumors have the potential to metastasize or circulate to other body regions as they become older. Ironically, the lymphatic system, which is the body's main mechanism for manufacturing and moving white blood cells and other cancer-fighting immune system cells throughout the body, is also the principal pathway of metastasis. White blood cells from the lymphatic system's immune system do not remove metastatic cancer cells, so these cells travel via the lymphatic capillaries and land in distant parts of the body where they might grow into new tumors and continue the disease process.

Breast cancer occurs often. Breast cancer is undoubtedly the terrifying sort of cancer diagnosis a person may get due to its well-publicized nature and propensity for death. However, it's important to remember that breast cancer is curable if found early on and given the appropriate care.

Breast cancer affects men and women equally. Although it happens less commonly in males than in women, breast cancer is still quite conceivable in men. While the majority of our talk will be on how breast cancer affects women, it should be highlighted that a lot of the material is equally relevant for males.

Chapter 1

Breast cancer: What is it?

Mutations, which are alterations in the genes that control cell development, are what lead to cancer. The cells may expand and divide thanks to the mutations uncontrollably.

Breast cancer is cancer that begins in breast tissue. Usually, breast cancer develops in the vents or lobules of the breast.

Milk is produced in glands called lobules, and ducts are the passageways that mesmerize milk from the glands to the nipple of the mammary gland. In addition to the fatty tissue and connective tissue found in the breast, cancer may also develop in the fatty tissue.

Cancer cells that are not under control will often infiltrate other healthy breast tissue and have the potential to spread to the lymph nodes located beneath the arms. Once cancer has spread to the lymph nodes, it is able to access a route that will allow it to spread to other areas of the body.

Indicators and manifestations of breast cancer

It is possible that breast cancer will not produce any symptoms in its early stages. In many instances, a tumor may not be large enough to be felt, but mammography will still reveal an anomaly if there is one.

If tumors can be felt, the first indicator is often the development of a lump in the breast that was not there before. On the other hand, not every lump is a sign of malignancy.
A wide range of symptoms may be present depending on the subtype of breast cancer. There is an increased degree of overlap between many of these symptoms, although some of them may be unique.

These are some of the most prevalent signs and symptoms of breast cancer:

- A new source of breast discomfort associated with a breast lump or tissue thickening that is distinguishable from the surrounding tissue.
- The skin on the breast that is red or discolored, pitted, and swollen; breast enlargement in whole or in part.
- A discharge from the nipple that is not breast milk.
- A bloody discharge coming from your
  nipple,
  peeling,
  scaling, or
  flaking of the skin on your nipple or breast,
- A rapid, inexplicable change in the shape or size of your breast,
- An inverted nipple changes the look of the skin on your breast.
- A mass or swelling that is located beneath your arm

Even if you experience one or more of these signs, however, it does not always signify that you have breast cancer. For example, a benign cyst might be the source of discomfort or a lump in your breast. Cysts can also produce breast lumps.

However, if you notice a lump in your breast or have other signs, you should make an arrangement with your doctor for additional testing and evaluation.

Different kinds of breast cancer
There are a number of subtypes of breast cancer, but generally speaking, they fall into one of two categories: invasive or noninvasive. Breast cancer that has not circulated to other parts of the breast is called breast cancer in situ.

Cancer that is noninvasive has not spread from the original tissue, in contrast to cancer that is invasive and has moved from the breast ducts or glands to other regions of the breast.

The following are the forms of breast cancer that fall under these two groups, which are the most frequent varieties of the disease:

Ductal cancer in situ. Ductal carcinoma in situ is a noninvasive situation. When you have DCIS, the cancer cells that are present in your breast are restricted to the ducts, and they have not yet spread into the surrounding breast tissue.

Lobular cancer in situ. LCIS stands for lobular carcinoma in situ, which refers to a kind of breast cancer that develops in the glands that produce milk. As is the case with DCIS, the cancer cells have not spread into the tissue that surrounds them.

Invasive ductal carcinoma. The most common kind of breast cancer is known as invasive ductal carcinoma or IDC for short. This particular subtype of breast cancer starts in the milk ducts of your breast and subsequently spreads to neighboring breast tissue. After the breast cancer has migrated to tissue that is outside of your milk ducts, it may start to spread to other neighboring organs and tissue. This can happen very quickly.

Invasive lobular carcinoma. The term "invasive lobular carcinoma" (ILC) refers to cancer that begins to form in the lobules of your breast and has spread to the surrounding tissue.

The following are some more, less frequent kinds of breast cancer:

Nipple Paget disease is a kind of Paget disease. This particular subtype of breast cancer begins in the venthole of the breast, but as it progresses, it starts to harm the skin and areola of the breast as well.

Phyllodes tumor. Connective tissue in the breast is the site of growth for this very uncommon subtype of breast cancer. The vast majority of these tumors are noncancerous, but a few of them are cancerous.

Angiosarcoma. This is a kind of cancer that develops in the breast and grows on the blood arteries or lymph vessels.

Your treatment choices and likely prognosis, in the long run, are both influenced by the sort of cancer you have.

Acquire additional knowledge about the many forms of breast cancer.

Breast cancer with an inflammatory component

Breast cancer with inflammation, often known as inflammatory breast cancer or IBC, is an uncommon yet aggressive subtype of breast cancer.

Because of this disorder, cells clog the lymph nodes that are located close to the breasts, which prevents the lymph arteries in the breast from draining normally. IBC does not result in the development of a tumor but rather causes the breast to enlarge, get red, and feel extremely heated. It's possible that your breast may seem wrinkly and lumpy, somewhat like an orange peel.

IBC is known to be very aggressive and has the potential to advance rapidly. Because of this, it is crucial that you make an appointment with your physician as soon as possible if you have any symptoms.

Breast cancer that is triple-negative

Another very uncommon kind of breast cancer is known as triple-negative breast cancer. According to the American Cancer Society, only around 10 to 15 % of breast cancer patients have this subtype of the disease (ACS).

A tumor must exhibit all three of the following features in order for a physician to make a diagnosis of triple-negative breast cancer:

- It does not have any estrogen receptors. These are the receptors on the cells that the hormone estrogen binds to, also known as attaches to. If a tumor has estrogen receptors, then estrogen has
the potential to encourage the growth of cancer.

- It does not include any progesterone receptors. These cells, known as receptors, are the ones that progesterone uses to connect to itself. When a tumor has progesterone receptors, the hormone progesterone has the potential to encourage the growth of the malignancy.

- It does not contain any extra proteins that operate as human epidermal growth factor receptor 2 (HER2) on its outside. A protein known as HER2 is responsible for the progression of breast cancer.

If a tumor satisfies all three of these requirements, a diagnosis of triple-negative breast cancer is made. This kind of breast cancer is characterized by a greater propensity for rapid growth and dissemination compared to other forms of breast cancer.

Because hormone treatment for breast cancer is ineffective in treating triple-negative breast cancer, the disease is notoriously difficult to treat.

Breast cancer is classified into phases by the size of the original tumor and the extent to which it has spread outside of the original site.

Cancers that are huge in size or that have spread to neighboring tissues or organs are considered to be at a more advanced stage than cancers that are still localized inside the breast. In order for physicians to stage breast cancer, they need to know the following:

Whether or not cancer has spread to neighboring tissue or organs, the size of the tumor,
whether or not the lump, and whether or not the cancer is invasive.

There are five primary stages of breast cancer, numbered from 0 to 4.
Breast cancer at its earliest stage
Stage 0 is DCIS. DCIS is characterized by the presence of cancer cells that have not migrated beyond the ducts of the breast into the surrounding tissue.

Breast cancer in its first stage

- Stage 1A. Less than two centimeters (cm) in width characterizes the initial tumor. There is no involvement of the lymph nodes.
- Stage 1B. Lymph nodes in the vicinity are affected by cancer. Either there is no tumor present in the breast, or the tumor is less than 2 centimeters in diameter.

Breast cancer in stage 2

- Stage 2A. Either the tumor is less than 2 centimeters in diameter and has only spread to one to three lymph nodes in the immediate area, or it is between 2 and 5 centimeters in diameter and has not migrated to any lymph nodes.
- Stage 2B. The tumor is between 2 and 5 centimeters in size and has circulated to between 1 and 3 lymph nodes in the axilla (the armpit), or it is more than 5 centimeters in size and has not migrated to any lymph nodes.

Breast cancer in its third stage

- Stage 3A.

It is possible that the cancer has progressed to between four and nine axillary lymph nodes or that it has increased the internal mammary lymph nodes. There is no set size for the main tumor.

The tumors are more than 5 centimeters in diameter. The malignancy has progressed to any of the breastbone nodes as well as one to three axillary lymph nodes.

- Stage 3B. There is evidence that a tumor has spread to the skin or chest wall, and it may or may not have circulated to up to 9 lymph nodes.
- Stage 3C. Cancer has spread to at least ten lymph nodes in the axilla, lymph nodes in the area of the collarbone, or internal mammary nodes.

Breast cancer in its fourth stage (metastatic breast cancer)

A woman with breast cancer in stage 4 may have a tumor of any size. Cancer cells from it have moved to lymph nodes both close and farther away, as well as to organs further away.

The tests that your physician does will establish the phase of your breast cancer, which will, in turn, influence the therapy that you get.

Chapter 2

What causes breast cancer

1. Alcohol

Consuming alcohol on a consistent basis is related to an increased likelihood of acquiring breast cancer.

If you consume alcohol, cutting down on how much you do so may help lower your chance of developing breast cancer.

2. Being overweight or obese

After menopause, a woman's chance of having breast cancer is increased if she has excess body fat, whether from being overweight or obese.

You may lessen your chances of anything bad happening by keeping a healthy weight.

3. Being physically active

Being physically active for around twenty minutes every day may help lower a woman's chance of developing breast cancer.

4. Cigarette smoking

There is mounting evidence to suggest that the risk of breast cancer is somewhat increased by smoking.

Women who have a severe breast cancer diagnosis in their family tree have a significantly increased risk.

When a woman starts smoking at a younger age, she puts herself in a more dangerous situation. Even after quitting smoking at least 20 years later, the higher risk will still be there.

Pregnancy and nursing are two different things.

Increasing a woman's family size may have a variety of effects on her chance of developing breast cancer.

Pregnancy, especially when carried to full term, is related to a lower incidence of breast cancer.

Breastfeeding your children has been shown to have a marginally protective effect against developing breast cancer.

5.   . Oral contraceptives and HRT

The capsule

Taking the combination oral contraceptive pill is associated with a marginally increased risk of developing breast cancer. However, after quitting for a few years, there is no longer any danger of this happening.

Replacement of hormones with hormone treatment (HRT)

While you are on HRT and for many years after you stop taking it, your chance of developing breast cancer is increased.

6.   Having a history of breast cancer in your family

Even if a member of your family has been diagnosed with breast cancer, it does not always guarantee that your own risk will rise. The majority of individuals do not have a high risk of developing breast cancer just because a close relative has been diagnosed with the disease.

However, if a person has a substantial history of breast cancer in their family, they have a greater chance of acquiring breast cancer themselves. This applies to both men and women.

7.   Myths

There are lots of misconceptions drifting around regarding what causes breast cancer.

For instance, some individuals are concerned that using deodorant or wearing a bra with underwires may raise their risk of breast cancer, although none of these behaviors really does so.

In a healthy organism, cancer cannot spread and cannot develop.

The stages of a normal, healthy cell's life cycle include growth, division, and, ultimately, death. A cell that is aberrant and does not follow this cycle is referred to as a cancer cell.

Cancer cells don't die off as they should but instead proliferate more aberrant cells that may infiltrate the tissue around them. They may also move to other sections of the body by traveling via the lymph system and the blood system.

Let's take a deeper look at what causes a normal cell to transform into a malignant cell, as well as the things that you can do to reduce the likelihood that you will acquire cancer.

Do all people have the potential to get cancer in their bodies?
No, not everyone has cancerous cells circulating in their body.

Our bodies are always creating new cells, and a small percentage of these cells have the potential to formulate into cancer. It's possible that at any one time,e we're making cells that already contain DNA damage, but it doesn't always guarantee those cells will develop into cancer.

The vast majority of the time, cells that have DNA damage either repair themselves or die off through a process called apoptosis. Only in the absence of either of those conditions is there a chance of developing cancer.

What sets cancer cells apart from other types of cells, such as normal cells?

In a nutshell, normal cells are ones that respond to instructions. Cancer cells don't.

The only time normal cells grow and divide is when they need to take the place of cells that have been damaged or that have aged. Mature cells are capable of performing specialized functions. When they have finished what they were meant to do, they pass away, thus completing their life cycle.

Cancer cells have genes that have been mutated and lack the specialized functions of normal cells. Cancer cells deviate significantly from the norm in their behavior. Whether or not they are required, they continue to proliferate and reproduce even after their numbers should have declined. Cancer is caused by abnormal cell growth that cannot be stopped.

Cancer cells congregate to form tumors, which then spread into the tissue in the surrounding area. These cells have the ability to splinter off and migrate to different regions of the body.

Cancer cells have the ability to alter the behavior of normal cells, further complicating the situation. They have the ability to stimulate healthy cells that are located close to them to develop new blood vessels, which helps cancerous tumors continue to receive the nutrients they require.

By preventing immune cells from telling cancer cells apart from other cells, cancer cells can frequently escape detection by the immune system.

What distinguishes cells that are benign from those that are malignant?

The difference between healthy cells and cancerous cells is quite significant.

Benign cells are noncancerous. They can occasionally overproduce and form tumors, but they are unable to invade other types of tissue even when they do so. In most circumstances, they do not pose a danger to a person's life, but this may change if the tumor becomes excessively large or presses against an organ. For instance, a benign brain tumor may still pose a threat to one's health.

When a benign tumor is removed, there is a low chance that it will return. There is no need for medication to be administered in order to prevent the return of benign cells since these cells do not spread.

Malignant cells are those that have the potential to cause cancer, which is a fatal disease. They are able to infiltrate neighboring tissues and propagate throughout the body once they get a foothold.

Any cells that are left behind after a malignant tumor is excised have the potential to trigger fresh growth. Because of this, cancer patients often need extra treatment in the form of chemotherapy, immunotherapy, or radiation therapy in order to locate and eliminate cancer cells located throughout the body.

What are some things you can take to lessen the possibility of developing cancer?

There is no way to totally remove the possibility of developing cancer. However, there are measures that may be taken to lower that possibility.

- **Avoid tobacco.** This covers cigars, cigarettes, pipes, and other smokeable and non-smokable forms of tobacco. Tobacco use is a contributing factor in one out of every two fatalities caused by cancer in the United States.
- **Get checked for cancer on a regular basis.** Screening procedures such as Pap smears and colonoscopies, for example, may discover abnormal cells in the body before they have the opportunity to transform into malignant cells. Other examinations, such as mammography, are able to identify cancer cells in a confined area before they begin to spread.
- **Consume alcohol, but do so in moderation.** Ethanol, which is included in alcoholic beverages, has been linked to an increased risk of formulating cancer over time. It is recommended that women have no more

than one drink of alcohol each day, while males may have up to two.

- **Be sure to shield your skin from the sun.** You can protect your skin from ultraviolet radiation by wearing protective clothing and using a broad-spectrum sunscreen. It is best to avoid the sun during the day and to steer clear of tanning beds and lights.
- **Maintain a diet that is both nutritious and balanced.** Make it a priority in your diet to consume a lot of fruits, vegetables, and grains that are whole. Reduce your consumption of sugary foods, processed meats, red meats, and processed meats.
- **Exercise**. The chance of developing cancer might be increased by a sedentary lifestyle. Every week, you should give yourself the goal of exercising for at least 150 minutes at a moderate intensity or 75 minutes at a strenuous intensity.

Have a discussion with your primary care physician about the possibility of receiving immunizations to help reduce the risk of certain malignancies.

Skin-to-skin contact is the primary mode of transmission for the sexually transmitted infection (STI) known as HPV. Cancers of the head and neck, sexual organs, and cervical region are all possible outcomes.

Hepatitis B, a viral illness that may lead to an increased risk of liver cancer, is also preventable by the use of a vaccination.

Discuss with your primary care physician about your risk for cancer and other preventative measures you may take to minimize that risk.

The bare essentials

Cancer cells are not present in the bodies of each and every one of us.

Because of the enormous number of cells that are continually being produced by your body, there is always the potential that some of them may get damaged. Despite this, there is still a chance that the injured cells will not develop into cancer.

Cancer is caused by damage to DNA, which may be passed down through families as a result of inherited genetic abnormalities or acquired from exposure to a substance in everyday life.

It is not possible to prevent genetic mutations from occurring, but adjusting some aspects of one's lifestyle, such as increasing the frequency of certain tests for cancer, may help reduce one's likelihood of having the disease.

Chapter 3

The treatment of breast cancer

Is there more than one kind of breast cancer?

Breast cancer comes in a wide variety of subtypes. Some are really hard to find. Your physician will be able to provide you with further information about the kind you have. The names of the most frequent kinds of breast cancer, as given in medical terminology, are listed below. (Cancer is sometimes referred to as carcinoma in certain circles.)

Ductal cancer in situ or DCIS

The term "very early breast cancer" refers to DCIS. In ductal carcinoma in situ or DCIS, the cancer cells are found solely inside the milk ducts. (The milk travels to the nipple via very small tubes known as ducts.) There is no evidence that cancer cells have made their way past the ducts' walls and into the surrounding breast tissue. DCIS can be treated in almost all women who have it.

Breast cancer has spread widely.

When breast cancer is said to be invasive, it signifies that cancer has spread beyond the original location where it began (for instance, a milk duct or milk gland) and is now invading (growing into) surrounding breast tissue. These malignancies have the potential to metastasize or circulate to other regions of the body. The vast majority of invasive breast cancers fall into one of these categories:

Invasive ductal carcinoma, often known as IDC, is the kind of breast cancer that occurs most frequently. It begins in one of the milk vents of the breast and then spreads throughout the surrounding breast tissue by growing through the wall of the duct.

This kind of cancer, known as invasive lobular carcinoma or ILC, begins in the milk glands, which are also referred to as lobules, and spreads into the breast tissue that is adjacent.

Inflammatory breast cancer (IBC) is a kind of cancer in which the Cancer cells block lymph arteries in the skin. The appearance of redness and a warm sensation on the breast surface are both caused by IBC. The skin may also have the appearance of being thick and pitted, much like the surface of an orange. The breast may grow larger, firmer, sensitive, or itching. IBC is not often accompanied by the sensation of a lump.

It's possible that an IBC won't show up on a mammogram since there aren't any lumps. This might make it more difficult to identify IBC in its early stages. It has a higher risk of metastasizing, and it is harder to treat than invasive ductal or lobular cancer.

Breast cancer that is triple-negative

TNBC is an assertive form of breast cancer that is resistant to a number of standard treatments. Because the cancer cells lack estrogen receptors, progesterone receptors, and another protein called HER2 that are tested for in breast cancers, this type of breast cancer is referred to as triple-negative. This is because the absence of these three types of proteins is one of the criteria used to classify breast cancers.

Proteins indicate that cancer may be more difficult to treat because there are fewer cure options available.

Concerns and inquiries to put to the physician

I'm curious as to why you think I have cancer.

Is there a possibility that I do not have cancer?

Could you jot down the name of the type of cancer you think I might have?

What steps will be taken after this?

How is it that my doctor has diagnosed me with breast cancer?

A change that appears on your mammogram could be the very first sign that you have breast cancer.

Alternatively, you might have discovered a lump or another change in your breast.

The doctor will examine you and then ask you questions about your health to get a better understanding of your condition. During the breast exam, the examiner will look for any changes in either the nipples or the skin of the patient's breasts. In addition, the doctor will examine the lymph nodes located above your collarbone and under your arm. If you have breast cancer and your lymph nodes are swollen or hard, this could indicate that cancer has spread.

More tests will be done on you if there are indications that breast cancer may be present.

The following are some of the possible examinations that you may need:

A mammogram is a kind of x-ray that is taken of the breast. Mammograms are often performed with the goal of detecting breast cancer in its early stages. On the other hand, you could have additional mammography to take a closer look at the potential issue with your breasts.
MRI scan: MRI machines provide detailed images without the use of x-rays by making use of radio waves and powerful magnets. MRIs are a useful tool for gathering information about the extent of the malignancy as well as searching for further cancers in the breast.

In breast ultrasound, a tiny tool that resembles a wand is pushed around on the patient's breast in a circular motion. It emits sound waves and is able to pick up the echoes produced when those sound waves reflect off of tissues. The echoes are converted into an image that is shown on the screen of a computer. The use of ultrasound may assist the physician in determining if a lump is a fluid-filled cyst, which does not often indicate cancer, or whether it is a solid mass, which may indicate malignancy.

undergoing a biopsy of the breast

A breast biopsy refers to the removal of a tiny amount of breast tissue by the doctor in order to examine it for any signs of malignancy. The only way for you to know for sure whether or not you have breast cancer is to have a biopsy performed.

There are a wide variety of biopsies to choose from. Inquire with your medical provider about the appropriate type for you. Every variety has both positive and negative aspects. The kind that you should use is determined by the nature of your situation.

It is sometimes necessary to do surgery to pull out all or part of the lump in order to determine whether or not the growth is cancerous. The hospital is the typical location for this procedure. You will get local anesthetic, which is the medicine that numbs the area, and you may also receive medication that puts you to sleep.

Examining for signs of the disease's progression in breast cancer

If breast cancer is detected, further tests, such as a CT (CAT) scan, PET scan, or bone scan, may be recommended to check for the disease's spread to other parts of the body. However, not every woman diagnosed with breast cancer has to undergo these tests.

Concerns and queries for the attending physician

What kinds of exams do I need to take?
Who exactly will administer these exams?
Where exactly will they be carried out?
Who can provide me with an explanation of the tests and the results?
What are the next steps that I need to take?

How severe is cancer in my body?

In the event that your biopsy sample contains breast cancer cells, those cells will be analyzed for specific proteins or genes that will assist in determining the most appropriate treatment for the condition.

Testing for proteins and genes

The breast cancer cells will be examined to see whether or not they have particular proteins known as estrogen and progesterone receptors. If the tumor has these proteins, the breast cancer is said to be positive for hormone receptors. In addition, the cells are examined to see whether or not the malignancy produces an abnormally high amount of the HER2 protein. If it occurs, the kind of cancer that results is known as HER2-positive. Because of the wide variety of medications that may be used to treat certain malignancies, the treatment process is sometimes simpler. It is referred to as triple-negative breast cancer if the tumor does not test positive for any of these proteins throughout the diagnostic process.

It is also possible to screen the cancer cells for particular genes, which may assist in determining whether or not chemotherapy might be beneficial and how likely cancer will return after treatment. Additional gene testing may assist in determining whether or not a particular medicine would be useful.

Inquire with your physician about the tests that will be performed and the possible interpretations of the outcomes.

The process of staging breast cancer

If you have breast cancer, the physician will want to determine how far the disease has spread from the original site. This technique is known as staging. In order to choose the most suitable course of therapy for you, your physician will first want to determine the stage of cancer you are battling.

The term "stage" refers to the degree to which cancer has progressed across the breast. In addition, it reveals if cancer has progressed to lymph nodes in the vicinity or to other organs that are located farther away in your body.
The stage of your cancer might be zero, one, two, three, or four. If the number is low, this indicates that cancer has not spread very far. A higher stage number, such as stage 4, indicates a more advanced and dangerous form of cancer that has spread beyond the breast. Make it a point to inquire with your physician about the stage of cancer and what it might entail for you.

Concerns and queries for the attending physician
Do you have any idea what stage the cancer is at?
In the event that this is not the case, how and when will you learn the stage?
Could you please clarify what the stage signifies in relation to my situation?
How severe is cancer in my body?
How long do you believe I'll live, taking into consideration the stage of cancer?

Are you aware of whether or not the following proteins are present in my cancer: the estrogen receptor, progesterone receptor, or HER2?

What exactly does it signify if any of these proteins are present in my cancer?

Is there a possibility that my cancer has undergone any gene mutations that might aid in the selection of medications for my treatment plan?

What will take place after this?

What kind of medical attention will I require?

There are a variety of therapies available for breast cancer.

Cancer in a particular area of the body may be treated by surgical removal and radiation therapy. They have no influence on the functioning of the rest of the body.

Drugs used in chemotherapy (often known as chemo), hormone treatment, targeted therapy, and immunotherapy may all reach cancer cells almost everywhere in the body.

When treating breast cancer, doctors often use more than one modality. The treatment strategy that is most suitable for you will be determined by the following factors:

The progression of the malignancy and its grade

If cancer possesses particular gene alterations or proteins, such as the HER2 protein or hormone receptors, then the cancer is more likely to spread.

The likelihood that a certain therapy will eradicate the disease or assist in its treatment in some manner. Your age

Any further health concerns that you have

Your thoughts and emotions towards the therapy, as well as the adverse consequences that it causes.

Surgical treatment of breast cancer

The vast majority of surgical procedures are performed on breast cancer patients who are women. Surgical procedures for the breast that are performed often include mastectomy, lumpectomy, and excision of lymph nodes from under the arm. Women who undergo breast surgery could also choose to have the breast form reconstructed, either at the same operation or at a later date. This decision might be made at any point in the process. The medical term for this procedure is "breast reconstruction."

A decision must be made between a lumpectomy and a mastectomy.

A lumpectomy removes the abnormal growth as well as a small portion of the surrounding normal breast tissue. It allows you to preserve a significant portion of your breast. The disadvantage is that you will almost certainly need radiation therapy after surgical procedures. However, after their mastectomy, some women may need to undergo radiation treatment.

Make sure you get all of the information before making a decision between a lumpectomy and a mastectomy. It's possible that, at first, you'll believe that having a mastectomy is the most effective approach to "get it all out." Because of this, the decision to get a mastectomy is made by some women. However, in most cases, having a lumpectomy followed by radiotherapy is equally as effective as having a mastectomy. Have a conversation with your cancer care team.

Gain as much knowledge as you can so that you may make the decision that is best for you.

Surgical procedures for reconstruction

If you are contemplating breast surgery, you should give some thought to the possibility of having your breast form recreated (breast reconstruction). This procedure is not intended to treat cancer. It creates a form for your breasts that is quite similar to the shape of your natural breast.

If you are considering having reconstruction after breast surgery, you should discuss your options with a plastic surgeon before the procedure is performed. It is possible that your breast will be able to be reconstructed either at the moment of surgery or at a later date.

Surgical complications may arise.

Any kind of surgical procedure has the potential for complications and dangers. Make sure to ask the doctor what kind of symptoms you should anticipate having. Please let your cancer maintenance team know if you have any difficulties following your operation. They need to be able to attend to you in resolving any issues that may arise.

Treatment with ionizing radiation

In order to eradicate cancer cells, radiation therapy makes use of high-energy rays (such as x-rays). After surgery, there is a possibility that some cancer cells may remain in the breast, chest, or armpit; this therapy may eliminate such cells. It is also effective in treating cancer that has circulated to other parts of the body outside the breast.

There are primarily two techniques to administer radiation:

A machine located on the outside of the body directs radiation toward the breast in the form of an external beam.

In brachytherapy, radioactive seeds are implanted directly into the breast tissue in the immediate vicinity of the malignancy.

Radiation therapy may have a variety of adverse effects.

In the event that your physician offers radiation therapy for you, it is important to discuss any potential adverse effects. The kind of radiation that was utilized determines the side effects. The following are the most prevalent adverse consequences of radiation exposure:

Alterations occur in the skin in the areas where radiation is delivered.

Feeling really exhausted (fatigued)

Most adverse effects become better once therapy finishes. Some may hold up better for longer. Have a conversation with the members of your cancer care team about what you may anticipate.

Chemo

Chemotherapy, which refers to the use of medications to treat cancer, is abbreviated as "chemo." The medications are either injected into a vein or taken orally, at which point they enter the bloodstream and are distributed throughout the majority of the body. It is possible to get chemotherapy either before, after, or both before and after surgical procedures.

Chemotherapy is often administered in cycles or rounds. After each session of the therapy, there will be a pause. The majority of the time, patients get two or more chemotherapy medicines simultaneously. The treatment may go on for a good number of months.

A side effect of chemotherapy

Chemotherapy may cause you to experience extreme fatigue, nausea, and hair loss. It can also make your stomach hurt. However, the majority of these issues are resolved after therapy is over.

The majority of chemo's negative effects are treatable in some manner. Be careful to let your cancer maintenance team know if you are undergoing any side effects so that they can assist you.

Treatment with hormones

Your body will continue to produce the female hormone estrogen until you go through the process of menopause. After that point, your body will continue to produce it, albeit in considerably lower quantities. Even in these minute doses, there is enough of a risk to increase the risk of breast cancer. Breast cancers like this may be treated with pharmaceuticals that either counteract the effects of estrogen or reduce the amounts of estrogen in the body. Hormone replacement treatment includes the use of medications like these.

Hormone therapy is another option that may be used to assist in reducing the likelihood of your cancer returning after it has been treated. In order to reduce the amount of estrogen in a woman who has already gone through menopause, she may be prescribed a medication known as an aromatase inhibitor. After surgery, one of these medications should be taken once every day for anywhere from five to ten years. Another medication known as tamoxifen is occasionally used as well. You do not need to have gone through menopause in order to utilize it; anybody may use it.

There are many additional medications that may help treat breast cancer, as well as other methods to reduce estrogen levels. Make sure to inquire about the possible side effects of any medication your doctor prescribes you.
Hormone replacement treatment may have adverse consequences.
Hot flashes and dryness of the vagina are the two negative effects of hormone treatment that women report experiencing the most often. There are remedies available for the majority of the negative effects that hormone treatment might cause. Be careful to let your cancer maintenance team know if you are undergoing any side effects so that they can assist you.

Drug treatment that is more specific
Certain forms of breast cancer, such as those that produce an abnormally high amount of the HER2 protein, are candidates for treatment with medications that belong to the targeted therapy category. These medications have a mostly negative effect on cancer cells and almost no effect whatsoever on normal cells in the body. They could be effective even if other treatments are unsuccessful. In general, they are accompanied by a distinct set of adverse effects than chemotherapy.

Negative implications of using targeted drugs in the treatment

Depending on the specific treatment that is administered, targeted pharmacological therapy for breast cancer may result

in a wide variety of unwanted side effects. Damage to the heart is a potentially major adverse effect that may occur with the use of medications that target the HER2 protein. Your physician will keep a careful eye on you to look for this and will routinely monitor your heart.

Immunotherapy

Immunotherapy is a kind of treatment that works by stimulating the body's natural immune system to wage war against breast cancer cells. These medications may either be administered intravenously or taken orally in tablet form.

Immunotherapy may sometimes have adverse consequences. Depending on the medicine that is used, immunotherapy might result in a wide variety of undesirable side effects. It is possible for immunotherapy medications to provoke a response when they are being administered intravenously to a patient. They may also lead the immune system to target other sections of the body that are healthy, which is a dangerous and even life-threatening adverse effect. During and after your therapy, your primary care physician will carefully monitor your progress.

Medical care is given during pregnancy.
In the event that you are pregnant and get a diagnosis of breast cancer, the therapy you receive will need careful planning. This is because you will want to receive the most effective treatment for your illness while simultaneously ensuring the

safety of your unborn child. Your oncology care team and your obstetrician (OB) will need to collaborate in order to

determine the appropriate therapy for you and when to provide it.
Have a discussion about the cure options available to you and your unborn child with both your obstetrician and your oncologist.

What about various other therapies that I have heard about?

When you have cancer, people may tell you about alternative treatments for either the illness itself or the symptoms it causes. These procedures may not always be considered the norm in medical practice. These therapies might consist of a variety of different items, such as vitamins, herbs, specific diets, and other things. It is possible that you have questions about therapies of this sort.
It is known that some of them are helpful, but the majority of them have not been examined. It has been displayed that some of them are not helpful, and a few of them have even been discovered to be hazardous. Consult your primary care physician before beginning usage of anything, including diet plans, vitamin supplements, or anything else.

Concerns and queries for the attending physician

What kind of therapy do you recommend for someone like me?
What precisely are we trying to achieve with this treatment?
Do you believe that it might perhaps cure cancer?

Will there be a need for surgical intervention? If such is the case, who will do the operation?
What exactly will the procedure entail?

Will I also need the use of other therapeutic modalities?
What are we trying to achieve with these treatments?
What potential adverse reactions can I have as a result of receiving these treatments?
What measures can I take to mitigate the potential adverse effects of this medication?
During the course of my therapy, will I be allowed to continue working?
How are we going to tell whether the therapy is really helping?
I was wondering if there was a clinical study in that I could participate.
What about the specialized diets and supplements that my coworkers keep telling me about? How am I going to determine whether they are risk-free?
What steps should I take to ensure that I am prepared for treatment?
Is there anything I can do to straighten up the efficacy of the therapy, and if so, what is it?
What Am I to do if I discover that I need assistance in traveling to my treatment appointments?
What are the following steps to take?
What may we expect after therapy is complete?

When therapy is over, you will feel relieved. You will continue to visit your oncologist for many years after your treatment for cancer has ended. Make it a point to attend each of these follow-up appointments. You will be subjected to physical examinations, blood tests, and maybe another test in order to differentiate whether or not the cancer has returned.

During the first few years of treatment, you may only need to come in once every few months. After a specific amount of time has been enacted after the completion of treatment, the frequency of follow-up appointments might decrease. You need to undergo a mammogram once a year if you .still have a breast. This is standard procedure. It is possible that you may require additional tests in addition to the therapy that you are receiving, such as frequent bone density tests or cardiac testing.

Having cancer and going through treatment may be challenging experiences, but they can also be opportunities to examine one's life in new and different ways. Talk to the people who are taking care of you for cancer to discover what you have to do to feel satisfied and how you can enhance your health if you are thinking about ways to do so.
You are unable to do anything about the fact that you have cancer. You have control over how you will spend the rest of your life, including whether or not you will make decisions that are good for your health and whether or not you will feel as well as you possibly can.

Chapter 4

The ten most important things to accomplish

- During treatment, here are some helpful hints for breast cancer patients
- Discover everything you have to know about your condition and the treatment options.
- At your appointments, bring a written list of the questions you have for your doctors so that you will get the best out of the moment you have with them.
- Make sure you get copies of your test findings and make sure you keep track of them in a notebook.
- Keep a list of questions that come up in between appointments so that you don't forget them, and be sure to take notes on the replies.
- Make sure that any choices you make are based on accurate information, and educate yourself as much as possible on both your diagnosis and treatment.
- Invest some time in finding the right doctor for you.

Specialists who treat breast cancer and work at cancer centers that are devoted to the disease provide patients with specialized knowledge and access to the newest medicines that are being tested in clinical trials. These types of institutions are able to provide various specialized services, such as physical therapy, dietary counseling, and social work, often all under one roof.

Get the necessary assistance for discussing your diagnosis with others around you. When you've been diagnosed with breast cancer, it may be just as challenging to tell your loved

ones and friends the news as it was for you to get the diagnosis from your doctor for the first time. It's possible that you're afraid of upsetting your family and friends or that you're anxious about how they'll respond to the situation. Even after you have told everyone the news, there will still be instances when you have trouble communicating in an open manner. Sometimes it's awkward to ask for assistance, answer queries about how you are doing, or tell well-meaning family and friends that you need some time and distance to yourself so that you can focus on getting well. Request a meeting with a social worker at your hospital, if one is available there, to talk about any emotional support or referrals to resources you may need. It's possible that participating in a local support group for breast cancer patients might also be of great assistance. Inquire at your local hospital or clinic about getting assistance in locating useful services in the surrounding region.

If you find yourself struggling with your finances, don't hesitate to ask for assistance. Your healthcare facility, whether it be a clinic or hospital, needed to have a social worker on staff, a patient navigator, or a financial services department in order to assist you in handling financial matters and interacting with private insurance companies, Medicare, and Medicaid. If you have concerns, seek an appointment.

Have a discussion with your primary care physician about managing the symptoms of menopause. Patients diagnosed with breast cancer who have been treated with chemotherapy, had their ovaries removed, or were forced to stop taking hormone replacement treatment at the time of their diagnosis

may have signs of menopause. Have a discussion with your primary care physician about the safest ways to treat menopause symptoms.

Eat well and stay healthy. The therapy you get for cancer may have an effect on your sense of smell and taste, as well as on your digestive process. During therapy, you may find that meals that you ordinarily love do not have a pleasant flavor, while, ironically, items that you do not often find appealing may taste more appetizing. Because you could like cooked veggies more than raw ones and be able to handle more of them, a vegetable stew or soup might appeal to you more than a salad would. If you eat smaller amounts of food more often throughout the day rather than three large meals each day, you may find that you have more strength and feel less nauseous. If you overindulge and go over your daily calorie limit, you run the risk of gaining weight. Increase your consumption of vegetables,
fruits,
whole grains,

nuts,
seeds, and legumes like black beans and lentils in order to aid in the battle against cancer. In order to accomplish a wide range of cancer-fighting nutrients, it is best to consume a variety of whole foods in a wide range of pigments (such as dark green for spinach, deep blue for blueberries, white for onions, and so on). During therapy, drinking alcohol is often not encouraged or suggested; nevertheless, if you want to drink, you should restrict your consumption to no more than three drinks per week. Recent research has shown a link

between drinking alcohol and an increased likelihood of developing breast cancer.

Take preventative measures to ward against lymphedema. The swelling of the soft tissues of the arm, hand, or chest wall that occurs as a result of lymphedema is a side effect that may occur during treatment for breast cancer. Even if it does not pose a danger to the patient's life, it must be treated immediately to stop it from deteriorating worse. There is a possibility that numbness, pain, and infection will accompany the swelling. There is no foolproof procedure for determining whether or not you are at risk for lymphedema; however, if you take the appropriate preventative measures, you may significantly lower your likelihood of acquiring the illness. In the event that you have symptoms, discuss the possibility of arranging physical therapy with your primary care physician or think about visiting a physical therapist even before the onset of symptoms in order to reduce the chance that you will experience them in the first place.

Get exercise. During therapy, light activity, like going for frequent walks, might help alleviate some of the emotional and physical side effects of the medication. After your therapy is finished, gradually increasing the amount of exercise you do will assist imprint improving tiredness and recovering the tone of your muscles. Increasing your circulation may also assist with chemobrain, which is a mental fogginess that some patients experience during and after chemotherapy treatment. Additionally, increasing your circulation may unquestionably boost both your mood and your perspective on life. You might

try activities such as yoga, tai chi, water aerobics, or swimming. Engage in some kind of physical activity for at least half an hour every day. Ask your doctor to direct you to a physical therapist if you are having trouble exercising or if you are unsure what to do if you are experiencing these issues.

Focus on maintaining strong bones. Maintaining bone health throughout your life is essential; b,t, if you are a female who has been diagnosed with breast cancer, maintaining bone health becomes even more essential. According to research, several therapies for breast cancer have been shown to cause bone loss. In addition, beyond the age of 50, the risk of osteoporosis developing in women is almost twice as high as the risk for males. Have a conversation with your heal healthcare about specific suggestions for maintaining healthy bones, such as taking calcium and vitamin D supplements and engaging in weight-bearing workouts that are suitable for your level of fitness.

Treatment as well as labor. During their course of treatment for cancer, some patients are able to continue working. However, it may be essential for certain people to cut down on their work capacity or perhaps take a vacation completely. It's possible that if you take some time off and then go back to work not long after your treatment is over; you'll find that it helps you keep your identity and even raises your self-esteem, not to mention that it increases your income. You should consider having a conversation with your employer about the possibility of pursuing other work arrangements, such as flextime, job sharing, or working from home. Options such as

these could make it easier for your mind and body to readjust to the requirements of your employment. As you transition back into your "regular" life, do your best to practice patience and focus on taking care of yourself.

The following list provides 12 foods that have been associated with fewer risk of breast cancer.

Foods that may reduce the chance of developing breast cancer

It is crucial to know that the development of breast cancer is linked to a wide variety of variables. Even while changing your food may help improve your overall health and lower your risk of cancer in general, this is just one piece of the cancer prevention jigsaw.

You still need to get regular breast cancer tests, such as mammograms and physical exams, even if you eat a diet that is high in nutrients. After all, discovery and diagnosis at an earlier stage considerably boost the chances of survival. Inquire with a qualified medical expert on the best breast cancer screening options.

Despite this, evidence shows that consuming certain foods may reduce the likelihood of developing the condition.

1. Leafy green veggies

These are just some of the leafy green vegetables that have been shown to have potential anti-cancer effects:

Kale
arugula
spinach mustard greens, chard

Carotenoid antioxidants
such as beta carotene,
Lutein, and zeaxanthin, may be found in vegetables that are dark green and leafy. Researchers have shown that women who have higher blood levels of certain antioxidants have a lower chance of developing breast cancer.

Women who had greater levels of carotenoids had a considerably decreased risk of breast cancer as compared to women who had lower levels of carotenoids. This was the conclusion of an earlier study that was conducted in 2012 and included eight studies and 7,011 women.
A similar finding was found in a major research that was conducted in 2015 that connected higher blood levels of total carotenoids to a decreased risk of breast cancer that ranged

from 18% to 28%, as well as a lower risk of recurrence and mortality in those who already had breast cancer. Over the course of twenty years, this research tracked 32,826 female participants.

The consumption of folate, which is a B vitamin that is rich in leafy green vegetables, has been observed in certain studies to be associated with a fewer danger of breast cancer. The research on whether the use of folate has a major influence, either positively or negatively, on the chance of developing breast cancer is equivocal. More research is required.

2. Cruciferous veggies

It's possible that eating cruciferous vegetables like broccoli, cabbage, and cauliflower will help reduce your likelihood of formulating breast cancer.
Compounds known as glucosinolates are found in cruciferous vegetables. Your body has the ability to convert them into molecules known as isothiocyanates. These have tremendous promise as anti-cancer agents.
Notably, research that included 1,493 Southern Chinese women found a relationship between greater overall consumption of cruciferous vegetables and a lower risk of breast cancer.

3. Allium veggies
Allium veggies include garlic, onions, and leeks, among others. They include a wide variety of minerals, including vitamin C, organosulfur compounds, and flavonoid antioxidants. There is a possibility that they have potent anti-

cancer effects. Researchers in Puerto Rico looked at the diets of 660 women and found that those who consumed more garlic and onions had a lower chance of developing breast cancer.

In a similar vein, research that was conducted in Iran and had 582 female participants indicated that high consumption of garlic and leeks might protect against breast cancer. Consuming a significant amount of raw onion may also provide some degree of protection. A high intake of cooked onion was also connected with an increased risk of breast

cancer, which is an intriguing finding that came out of the research.

Therefore, there is a need for more studies on the subject of onions and breast health.

4. Citrus fruits

Citrus fruits include:

oranges\grapefruits

lemons

limes\stangerines

Substances that may protect against breast cancer may be found in abundance in citrus fruits and the peels of those fruits. These compounds include:

Flavonoids such as quercetin, hesperetin, and naringenin flavonoid antioxidants such as folate and vitamin C carotenoids such as beta-cryptoxanthin and beta carotene flavonoid

The antioxidant, anti-inflammatory, and anti-cancer properties of these nutrients have been shown.

Citrus fruits have been linked to a lower risk of formulating many types of cancer, including breast cancer, according to a study. A previous literature analysis from 2013 that included six trials and 8,393 persons found that high consumption of citrus was associated with a 10% lower risk of breast cancer.

5. Berries

Consuming berries on a regular basis has been shown to reduce the chance of developing various malignancies, including breast cancer.

Antioxidants found in berries, such as flavonoids and anthocyanins, have been demonstrated to protect against cellular damage and the growth and spread of cancer cells. Flavonoids and anthocyanins are also among the antioxidants found in berries.

Notably, a research review published in 2013 that included 75,929 female participants found a correlation between greater consumption of berries, and blueberries in particular, with a reduced risk of estrogen receptor-negative breast cancer.

6. Grapes, peaches, apples, and pears, among other fruits

It has been shown that eating fruits, particularly peaches, apples, pears, and grapes, may reduce one's risk of developing breast cancer.
Women who took at least two servings of peaches per week had up to a 41% lower chance of developing estrogen

receptor-negative breast cancer, according to the results of the major research that was published in 2013 and was noted above.

Polyphenol antioxidants from peaches, according to earlier research conducted in 2014, were shown to limit the development and spread of a human breast cancer cell line that had been implanted in an animal model. This finding is rather interesting.

Intake of apples and pears has also been associated with a reduced danger of breast cancer, according to research that analyzed data from hundreds of thousands of women.

Flavonoids and anthocyanins are two examples of the types of substances that have been isolated from grapes and shown to be effective in inhibiting the growth of breast cancer cells in test tubes. There is a need for more study with human subjects.

7. Fish rich in lipids

The amazing health advantages of fatty fish, such as salmon, sardines, and mackerel, have brought to their widespread consumption. There is some evidence that the omega-3 fats, selenium, and antioxidants included in certain foods, notable astaxanthin, may give some protection against cancer.

A number of studies have indicated that consuming fish high in fat may particularly lower the chance of developing breast cancer.

One older literature review was published in 2013, and it looked at 21 studies that involved a total of 883,585 participants. According to the results of a current study, women who consume the greatest amounts of omega-3s from seafood have up to a 14% lower chance of developing breast cancer compared to those whose omega-3 consumption is the lowest.

Similar conclusions have been reached in other research on the topic of eating fish and the fatty acids it contains.
It is possible that reducing the number of refined oils and ultra-processed foods you consume, together with increasing the amount of fatty fish you consume, can help you lower your chance of developing breast cancer.

8. Foods that are fermented

Probiotics and other nutrients may be found in fermented foods such as
yogurt,
kimchi,
miso, and sauerkraut. These foods have been shown to lessen the risk of breast cancer.
Consumption of dairy products, especially fermented dairy products like yogurt and kefir, was associated with a lower chance of breast cancer, according to a literature analysis that was conducted in 2015 and included 27 separate research.
Research conducted on animals and in test tubes both points to the possibility that the immune-boosting properties of specific probiotics are responsible for this protective effect.

9. Beans

Fiber, vitamins, and minerals may all be found in abundance in beans. In particular, the high fiber content of these foods may provide some protection against breast cancer.

According to the discoveries of research that included 4,706 women, a high diet of beans was shown to lower the incidence of breast cancer by up to 20% compared to a low intake of beans.

In addition, research that included 1,260 Nigerian women found that those who ate beans the most had a risk of breast cancer, which was up to 28% lower than those who ate the fewest beans. This finding was compared to those who ate the fewest beans.

10. Aromatic plants and seasonings

There is some evidence that the plant components found in herbs and spices may help protect against breast cancer. Vitamins, fatty acids, and antioxidants called polyphenols are included in this category.

Carvacrol and rosmarinic acid are two examples of powerful antioxidants that may be found in oregano. According to the findings of research conducted in 2017 using test tubes, these antioxidants had strong anti-cancer benefits when used against aggressive breast cancer cell lines.

Apigenin, a flavonoid that is prevalent in parsley, and curcumin, the primary active ingredient in turmeric, have both been shown to possess strong anti-cancer activities. Both of these flavonoids have been found in turmeric.

It is recommended that you incorporate a broad range of herbs and spices in your diet, such as thyme, curry spice mixtures, and ginger, since many additional herbs and spices, in addition to these, have potent anti-cancer properties.

11. Whole grains

Whole grains, such as wheat, barley, barley, quinoa, and rye, are very high in a number of essential elements, including fiber, vitamins, minerals, and antioxidants.

In addition to that, there is a possibility that they offer potent anti-cancer effects.

Research that was conducted in 2016 indicated that women who consumed at least seven servings of whole grains on a weekly basis had a considerably decreased chance of developing breast cancer. [Citation needed] [Citation needed]

Eating a greater quantity of carbohydrates of high quality, such as whole grains, was connected with a lower chance of getting breast cancer over 12 years, according to the findings of another research that included 10,812 middle-aged women as participants.

In addition, other evidence shows that consuming a diet that includes whole grains may help protect against a number of other cancers, including pancreatic, colorectal, stomach, and esophageal cancers.

12. Walnuts

Walnuts offer a lengthy list of advantages and are a fantastic source of heart-healthy fats, including alpha-linolenic acid. Walnuts can be found in most grocery shops and health food stores.

It is fascinating to note that some studies indicate that including walnuts and other kinds of nuts in one's diet may even help reduce the risk of developing breast cancer.

Those participants in a study that involved 201 people and was conducted in 2015 found that those participants who consumed the highest amount of walnuts,

peanuts,

and almonds each week had a risk of developing breast cancer that was two to three times lower than those participants who didn't consume any nuts.

In a second, more limited trial, the effects of eating walnuts on breast cancer patients were investigated. The study discovered that eating walnuts on a daily basis for two to three weeks led to substantial changes in the levels of particular

genes that drive the development and spread of breast cancer cells. One serving of walnuts is equal to 57 grams (about 2 ounces).

In addition, test-tube research that was conducted in 2016 showed that certain chemicals that were extracted from walnuts have the ability to inhibit the development of breast cancer cells by 63 percent.

Conclusion

A comprehensive strategy for preventing, detecting, diagnosing, and treating cancer should always be included as an essential part of any such strategy. Its primary objective is to alleviate the suffering of cancer patients by curing them or significantly extending their lives, all while preserving their quality of life. It is imperative that a diagnosis and treatment plan are never produced in a silo if the plan is to have any chance of being successful. It is essential that it be connected to an early detection program so that cases may be identified at an early stage when a cure is more likely to be successful and there is a better possibility of recovery. It also needs to be combined with a palliative care program in order to provide patients with advanced cancers who are no longer able to benefit from treatment with adequate relief from their physical, psychosocial, and spiritual suffering. Patients with advanced cancers are patients who can no longer benefit from treatment. In addition, programs should include a component for raising awareness in order to educate patients, family members, and members of the community about the factors that increase the risk of developing cancer, as well as the necessity of taking preventative measures to reduce the risk of developing cancer.

In situations where there are few resources, the primary focus of cancer diagnostic and treatment services should be on people who appear with tumors that are treatable, such as breast, cervical, and oral cancers that may be discovered in their early stages. They may also include pediatric acute lymphocytic leukemia, a kind of cancer that has a great possibility for treatment despite the fact that it cannot be diagnosed in its early stages. First and foremost, it is essential that services be delivered in a fair and environmentally responsible way. If and when more resources become available, the initiative may be expanded to encompass not just diseases that can be cured but also tumors for which therapy can significantly increase patients' chances of surviving the disease.

9 798369 819487